Mechanical Ventilation Made Easy

by Michael Fischer

CHECK OUT OTHER TITLES BY THIS AUTHOR AT:

WWW.MICHAELFISCHERAUTHOR.COM

Contents

Introduction to Mechanical Ventilation

History

Respiratory and mechanical ventilation are perhaps the most important aspects of patient care existing today. In ACLS and BLS, the ABCs are drilled into your mind. Respiratory is two-thirds of the ABCs (airway and breathing). Even in the Bible, the significance of the airway is discussed. Genesis 2:7 (KJV) states, "And the Lord God formed man of the dust of the ground and breathed into his nostrils the breath of life, and man became a living soul." So when you really think about it, the respiratory profession is the oldest recorded.

Paracelsus (1493 – 1541) is credited with creating the first form of mechanical ventilation when he placed a tube into a patient's mouth and ventilated the patient with fireplace bellows.

Andreas Vesalius (1514 – 1564) was the first person to have placed a reed or cannula into the trachea of an animal and blow into it.

Robert Hooke (1635 – 1703) was a member of a prominent academic group, The Royal Society, in London. In this group, Hooke was involved in many experiments, including the use of bellows to keep an animal alive while the thorax was opened.

In 1767, the Dutch formed the Society for the Rescue of Drowned Persons. Their most notable contributions included the use of mouth-to-mouth resuscitation as well as chest compressions.

In 1871, Friedrich Trendelenburg, a surgeon, introduced the first cuffed tube used in preventing aspiration during surgery of the larynx.

In 1911, Dräger developed the pulmotor, an artificial breathing device used by fire and police units for resuscitation.

The polio epidemic of the 1950s brought on the rapid advancement of negative pressure ventilation. Although forms of it have been in existence since the mid-1800s, it took a medical crisis to put urgency on the matter. Negative pressure ventilation, most commonly found in "the iron lung," was a process in which a patient was placed in a chamber that covered the chest and abdomen. The chamber would allow ventilation to occur through the creating of a negative pressure outside of the chest. This negative pressure would transfer through to the thoracic cavity, causing air to move into the lungs. The biggest drawback of this form of ventilation was that there was no access to the patient's chest for a physical exam.

Positive pressure ventilation, as described earlier through the works of Paracelsus, has been slowly developing throughout history and is the primary method used to ventilate today. It is for this reason that the remainder of this text discusses the modes of positive pressure ventilation.

Definitions

The world of medicine has a language all its own. We have medical terms, lingo, and abbreviations that may have some outsiders believing that they have entered into a foreign country. Mechanical ventilation is no different. Sometimes when we teach about mechanical ventilation, we overload our students with definitions and abbreviations so much so that it hampers their ability to grasp the basics. Before I get started, you will need to understand and become familiar with the "basic" definitions and abbreviations used in the following chapters.

Barotrauma: Damage to the lungs caused by high pressure or high volume.

Compliance (C_L): A measurement of the lungs' ability to expand.

F_IO_2: The percentage of oxygen delivered to the patient.

Minute ventilation: The amount of air breathed in and out in one minute. This is calculated as respiratory rate X tidal volume.

Peak inspiratory pressure (PIP): The highest pressure measured in the lungs upon inspiration.

Positive end expiratory pressure (PEEP): A maneuver that maintains the patient's airway pressure above baseline. PEEP helps to maintain recruited alveoli and is measured in cm H_2O.

Plateau pressure (P pl): The measurement of pressure applied to the small airways and alveoli during inspiration. Plateau pressure is measured during a period when no gas flow is entering the lungs (a static condition). This is done by adding an inspiratory pause of 0.5 to 1 second after peak inspiratory pressure is achieved. This pressure can also reflect how easily the alveoli can be distended.

Pneumothorax: A hole in the lungs which leads to air or gas entering into the pleural space of the thorax. This condition can lead to lung collapse.

Pressure support: An amount of pressure measured in cm H_2O delivered to a patient during a spontaneous inspiration.

Respiratory rate (r.r. or breaths/minute): The number of breaths a person takes or receives from the ventilator in one minute.

Tidal volume (V_T): The amount of air breathed in or out during a single breath.

Physiology

The Respiratory Cycle:

To understand how best to use a ventilator, you must first understand some basic principles about how you breathe.

Air moves from an area of high pressure to an area of low pressure. This difference in pressure is called a pressure gradient. Therefore, to have air outside of the body move into the lungs, a pressure gradient must occur. This pressure gradient is caused by thoracic expansion and contraction.

We often think of breathing as just an in-and-out phase when, in fact, there are four phases of the respiratory cycle.

Phase 1: Beginning of inspiration:

The respiratory muscles begin to contract, causing the thorax to expand. This process creates a negative pressure in the airways, and air begins to enter the lungs.

Phase 2: End inspiration:

The respiratory muscles have stopped contracting during this phase. As the atmospheric pressure equilibrates with the lung pressure, inspiration stops.

Phase 3: Beginning of exhalation:

As the respiratory muscles relax, the pressure in the lungs becomes greater than the atmospheric pressure. At this point, air exits the lungs back into the atmosphere.

Phase 4: End exhalation:

The pressure in the lungs is equal to the atmospheric pressure (the air pressure that exists outside of the body). Air does not move either into or out of the lungs during this phase.

Now that you have an understanding of the ventilation phases, I will describe how mechanical ventilation plays a role during each phase.

Phase 1: Beginning of inhalation:

In mechanical ventilation, this phase is called the triggering mechanism. There are four ways in which the ventilator can be triggered to begin inspiration: pressure, flow, time, or volume.

Pressure-triggered: ventilation came about when it was determined that patients may want to take a spontaneous breath, which is also known as assisted ventilation. The operator sets the pressure sensitivity on the ventilator. As the patient attempts to take a breath, they create a negative pressure against the circuit. When the set pressure is reached, the ventilator will begin the breath.

Flow-triggered: inspiration requires a ventilator that has the ability to sense inspiratory flow from the patient. Many old style ventilators do not have this capability. For the newer ones that do have this feature, the inspiration begins when the ventilator senses a drop in the circuit flow, which is caused by the spontaneous inspiratory effort from the patient.

Time-triggered: ventilation is also called controlled ventilation. In this mode, the patient cannot cycle a breath. The ventilator/operator sets or controls the respiratory rate. If the rate is set at 12 times per minute, then the ventilator will cycle a breath every 5 seconds.

Volume-triggered: inspiration from the ventilator begins when a preset volume is reached on a spontaneous effort from the patient.

Neurologically triggered: the inspiratory phase begins when a neurological impulse from the brain is read from a NAVA catheter. The NAVA catheter is essentially an NG tube with electrodes at the end that sit at the level of the diaphragm. These electrodes pick up the same neurological impulse that the diaphragm receives via the phrenic nerve from the brain.

Phase 2: End Inspiration:

This phase is also known as the cycling method. As in the beginning of inspiration, the ending of inspiration can be pressure-cycled, flow-cycled, time-cycled, or volume-cycled.

Pressure-cycled: Inspiration will stop when a preset pressure is reached within the patient circuit. The tidal volume that the patient will receive will be variable. It will change based on the patient's compliance, inspiratory time, and flow pattern. In cases where a larger circuit leak is present, the preset pressure may never be reached. Therefore, the inspiratory phase will not stop, and the patient will not receive an adequate tidal volume.

Time-cycled: This cycle occurs when you are able to set the inspiratory time on the ventilator. When the inspiratory phase reaches this set time, the ventilator will begin the expiratory phase. In time-cycled ventilation, the flow, tidal volume, and pressure will be variable. If you have a set tidal volume, as in volume control ventilation, with a set inspiratory time of one second, then the ventilator needs to push this amount of air into the lungs during this set time. The higher the tidal volume, the greater the flow of gas will need to be to reach the goal. The peak inspiratory pressure will also be limited. It will take a greater amount of pressure to push the air into the lungs if the inspiratory time is not long enough. If you have a set pressure to achieve rather than a tidal volume, then the volume the patient will receive is going to be variable. If you have the set pressure at 20 cm H_2O with an inspiratory time of one second, you will give the patient a greater tidal volume than if the inspiratory time was only .75 seconds.

Volume-cycled: Inspiration will stop when a preset volume is reached. The inspiratory pressure will be variable and is primarily dependent on the patient's lung condition. If the lungs are stiff or non-compliant, it will take a greater amount of pressure to deliver the volume than on a patient with healthy lungs, which are easily expandable.

PHASES 3 AND 4: End of Exhalation and Beginning of Inspiratory Phase

I will combine these two phases into what is called the expiratory phase. During the exhalation phase, air moves out of the lungs and returns to the expiratory side of the ventilator. Most of the newer ventilators on the market today possess microchip technology, which provides the ability to measure the volumes returned from the patient. It is important to measure the exhaled volumes to see if they match the inspired volumes. If the volume coming back from the patient is less than what was delivered, then you need to diagnose the problem. Some of the most common problems are:

- Circuit disconnect on the expiratory side
- Expiratory time is not long enough, creating air trapping or auto PEEP
- Expiratory filters may be saturated with moisture, therefore not allowing the flow of air to pass through to the ventilator

During the exhalation phase, the weight of the chest and the natural tendency of the respiratory muscles to relax will allow for the exhalation to occur. The pressure gradient that now exists between the lungs and the atmospheric air will also play a factor in the exhalation process. When mechanically ventilating a patient, the primary factor for stopping exhalation is time. Most modes of ventilation have a set respiratory rate with a set inspiratory time, thus automatically setting the expiratory time. For example, if you have a set respiratory rate of 12 breaths per minute with a one second inspiratory time, then you will have a 4 second expiratory time.

60 seconds ÷ 12 bpm = 5 seconds

5 seconds – 1 second inspiratory time = 4 seconds' expiratory time

In modes where there is no set respiratory rate, such as pressure support or volume support, the patient will spontaneously begin the next inspiratory cycle, thus ending the expiratory phase.

PEEP is another factor that affects the expiratory phase. PEEP (Positive End Expiratory Pressure) is a set amount of pressure existing in the ventilator circuit during the exhalation phase. This pressure transfers from the circuit to the patient's airways and will keep the alveoli somewhat distended during exhalation. PEEP prevents partial or complete collapse of the airways during exhalation, thus creating a greater inspiratory pressure to open these airways. Again, if there is not enough time for a patient to fully exhale before the next breath begins, air trapping or auto PEEP may occur. The air that did not have time to exit the lungs remains and creates its own amount of pressure against the alveoli. This pressure is called auto PEEP and will not allow the alveoli to collapse completely.

Since you have determined that PEEP can be good, you may be asking what is so bad about auto PEEP? PEEP and auto PEEP need to be managed carefully. There can be detrimental effects to having excessive PEEP. Primarily, too much PEEP can transfer this pressure against the vessels of the heart and can lead to a decreased blood pressure. It is very important to monitor the patient's blood pressure when administering PEEP.

Resistance

Airway resistance is the impedance or opposition to the flow of gas. The airway resistance equation is:

$$R = \frac{\Delta P}{v} = \frac{Patm - Pa}{v}$$

R = Resistance
ΔP = Change in Pressure
V = Volume

Patm = Atmospheric Pressure
Pa = Alveolar Pressure

Normal airway resistance is 0.6 to 2.4 cm H_2O/L/Sec.

We must discuss the two types of flow in order to fully understand all aspects of airway resistance: laminar flow and turbulent flow. Water flowing through a pipe is experiencing laminar flow, while water flowing through a rocky riverbed is experiencing turbulent flow. The same principle applies to your airways.

Reynolds number is an equation developed by Osborne Reynolds, a British engineer and physicist, and is useful in determining if the flow of gas is smooth (laminar) or rough (turbulent).

Reynolds number: $N_R = \frac{v \, X \, d \, X \, 2r}{\eta}$

v = Velocity
d = Density
r = Radius
□ = Viscosity

Reynolds number of < 2000 represents laminar flow, while a number > 2000 represents turbulent flow.

Poiseuille's law describes the physical attributes of laminar flow and puts it into an equation:

$R = 81\square / ^{\pi}r^{4}$

R = Resistance
l = Length of Tubing
r = Radius of Tubing

In laminar flow, the radius of the tubing will have a greater effect than any other factor in the above equation. Based on Poiseuille's law, if you double the size of the tubing, or in this case the airway, you will decrease the resistance by a factor of 16, while a decrease in the airway by one-half will cause a 16-fold increase in resistance.

Turbulent flow does not have an equation like that of laminar flow. Go back to the example of water flowing through a rocky riverbed. Various factors affect the flow of the water: the size of the rocks, the number of rocks, other debris that may exist, and living organisms within the water. The human airway is similar to the riverbed when it comes to understanding how turbulent flow works. Flow is affected by the structures of the upper airways, such as the turbinate bones in the nasal passageway or even the hairs of the nose (vibrissae). It may also be affected by: secretions; obstructions, such as aspirated food; and natural bifurcations of the airways. The more obstructions present, the greater the resistance to the flow.

Treating airway resistance is, for the most part, quite simple. In the case of laminar resistance, it is simply a matter of increasing the size of the airway. This can be done by changing the endotracheal tube to a larger size or by the delivery of a bronchodilator to increase the diameter of the anatomical airways. Turbulent resistance may be corrected by: suctioning chest percussion, adding humidification, and the use of heliox (a low-density gas mixture of oxygen and helium).

Modes of Mechanical Ventilation

As you are well aware, there are many modes of mechanical ventilation, but I will be covering only the basic modes. Many other advanced modes exist, yet they would require more extensive analysis. My goal is to give you a firm foundation on which to build, and building on a shaky foundation yields an unstable structure as teaching advanced technique before the basics are fully understood yields an unstable education.

I will begin with the modes that provide the most support to the patient and work through to the modes in which the patient is doing most of the work. It is also important to understand that I am teaching the basics of mechanical ventilation. After completing this book, your goal should be to know and understand the following:

- Definitions of basic mechanical ventilation
- Abbreviations used in basic mechanical ventilation
- Modes of basic mechanical ventilation
- Normal blood gas values
- Basic ventilator changes to correct out-of-range blood gas values

Reading and understanding this book is *not* enough knowledge for you to make ventilator changes on your own. You must always follow the clinical practice guidelines established by the facility at which you are employed. Now, let's get started!

Controlled Mechanical Ventilation (CMV)

This mode is rarely used today. When you see the word "control" used in describing a mode of ventilation, it means that *you* are taking control, not the patient. In controlled mechanical ventilation, the ventilator takes total control of the patient's breathing. You will enter a set tidal volume and set respiratory rate. What you set is what the patient receives with every breath. Any effort by the patient to breathe above the set rate will be ignored. An example of typical settings is as follows:

Tidal volume:	500 ml
Respiratory rate:	12 breaths/minute
F_IO_2:	40 %
PEEP:	5 cm H_2O

Your patient will receive a tidal volume of 500 ml, 12 times per minute, for a minute ventilation of 6.0 liters (tidal volume x respiratory rate = minute ventilation). This mode is appropriate if the patient is paralyzed by medications and there is no chance of the patient making any inspiratory effort. If the patient does make an effort, that effort will be ignored by the ventilator, and the patient may begin fighting with the ventilator.

Volume Control

You may have also heard this mode termed *assist-control.* As in controlled mechanical ventilation, you will again set a tidal volume and respiratory rate for your patient. However, this time, when the patient takes a spontaneous breath above the set respiratory rate, they will receive the same tidal volume delivery that was delivered during a controlled breath. An example of typical volume control settings are as follows:

Tidal volume:	500 ml
Respiratory rate:	12 breaths/minute
F_IO_2:	40%
PEEP:	5 cm H_2O

As you can see, the settings arc the same as in the CMV mode. Based on these settings, the patient will receive a controlled breath of 500 ml at least 12 times per minute. If the patient is breathing greater than 12 times per minute, then *each additional breath the patient takes will also be controlled.* The ventilator will deliver 500 ml for each of the spontaneous breaths.

The main advantage of volume control is that it guarantees the patient will receive a set tidal volume and respiratory rate. This means the patient will also receive set minimum minute ventilation. One of the disadvantages of this mode is that although we have a guaranteed tidal volume, the peak inspiratory pressure will vary. If the patient's lungs become stiff and less compliant, the peak inspiratory pressure will rise. This can be dangerous to the patient unless you have set the peak inspiratory alarm at a safe level. The peak inspiratory alarm allows the ventilator to terminate the breath if the peak inspiratory pressure delivered to the patient reaches the limit you have set on the alarm. Nevertheless, even causing a single breath at a high peak inspiratory pressure may cause damage to the patient's lungs. An example of this damage may be barotrauma or possibly a pneumothorax.

Pressure-Regulated Volume Control (PRVC)

Notice the word "control" appears again in this mode. PRVC is considered by some to be the best of **Pressure Control**

"Control" is, again, the key word in this mode. The ventilator is still taking complete control of the patient's breathing. The key difference between pressure control and volume control is simply how the breath will be delivered. In volume control, you set a certain tidal volume to be delivered with each breath as the peak inspiratory pressure varies. In pressure control, you set a peak inspiratory pressure to be delivered with each breath, and the volume will now vary.

An example of typical pressure control settings are as follows:

Peak pressure:	24 cm H_2O
Respiratory rate:	12 breaths/minute
F_IO_2:	40%
PEEP:	5 cm H_2O

The patient on these settings will now receive 12 breaths per minute. On each inhalation, the machine will deliver a breath until 24 cm H_2O is achieved. At that time, the inspiration will stop. Depending on the compliance of the lungs, the amount of volume the patient receives will vary. If the patient is 60 years old, overweight, and has a severe case of pneumonia, then 24 cm H_2O will deliver a far smaller tidal volume than a patient who is 20 years old, has never smoked, and runs two miles every day.

The main advantage of pressure control is safety. It does not matter how poor the compliance of the lungs becomes since each breath will always terminate at the set peak inspiratory pressure. The chance of barotrauma occurring is far less than in volume control. A drawback to pressure control is that it does require more careful monitoring of the patient because, as lung compliance changes, so will the returned tidal volume. Therefore, there is no guaranteed tidal volume or minute ventilation. As lung compliance changes, the respiratory therapist must adjust the set peak pressure in order to keep up with the new demands of the patient. If these changes are not carefully watched, the patient could easily become either over ventilated or under ventilated.

An example of how a patient can be affected by each mode of ventilation might help to explain the differences further. Let us say a patient is rolled onto their side while the nurse is changing the linens. While the patient is rolled over, a mucus plug occludes the left lung. All you are ventilating now is the right lung. In the volume control setting that was previously illustrated, the right lung will now receive the entire tidal volume of 500 ml. This high volume will create a high peak inspiratory pressure, and in just one breath you may have caused significant damage to the airways. Using the same illustration, the patient in pressure control will receive the same peak inspiratory pressure of 24 cm H_2O to the right lung, which is the same amount of pressure delivered before. The patient might be under ventilated until the plug is removed. However, a patient can go quite some time being under ventilated before any harm can occur, while just one breath set at too high of a pressure can be damaging.

Here is another example: after suctioning a patient, the compliance of the lungs has now increased. For the patient in volume control, this means each delivered breath will still be at a tidal volume of 500 ml, but the peak inspiratory pressure needed to achieve this volume has gone down. For the patient in pressure control, the same peak pressure is still being delivered; however, the tidal volume received by the patient has now increased due to the increased compliance of the lungs.

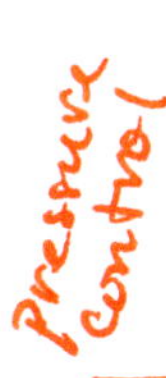

both worlds, combining volume control and pressure control ventilation. When you put a patient on PRVC, as in volume control, you are going to set a tidal volume and respiratory rate. The first breath the machine delivers will be a volume breath delivering the tidal volume you set. The ventilator will measure the plateau pressure used in delivering the initial volume breath as a pressure-controlled breath. *The ventilator will adjust the amount of pressure to deliver to the patient by measuring returned volumes and automatically adjusting the pressure based on those returns.* The change will be in increments of 3 cm H_2O per breath. The maximum peak pressure that will be delivered will be no more than 5 cm H_2O below the set high-pressure alarm. The basic settings for this mode will be the same as in volume control:

Tidal volume:	500 ml
Respiratory rate:	12 breaths/minute
F_IO_2:	40%
PEEP:	5 cm H_2O

Based on these settings, the first breath delivered will be a volume breath of 500 ml. Let us assume the plateau pressure measured in this breath is 24 cm H_2O. The next breath will now be a pressure-controlled breath delivering a breath at 24 cm H_2O. Now, each breath the patient receives will be a pressure breath above the set rate, and the breath is delivered at the set pressure of 24 cm H_2O.

Going back to the scenario used earlier in which one side of the lungs is plugged using the PRVC mode, the right side will still receive only 24 cm H_2O. The volume returned will more likely be a smaller volume as you are only receiving volume from the right side. The next breath will be delivered at 27 cm H_2O. Each additional breath will increase by 3 cm H_2O until the desired volume is achieved or when you have reached a peak inspiratory pressure of 5 cm H_2O below the set high peak pressure alarm. You still run a risk of inducing barotrauma if the condition is not corrected quickly or if the high-pressure alarm is set too high.

Adaptive Support Ventilation (ASV)

The concept of ASV is based on “the least work of breathing” model by Otis in the 1950s. It is a dual-controlled mode that switches from a control type of mode to a SIMV or pressure support type of mode based on the patient’s status.

Upon setup, the clinician will input the following information:

- Patient’s ideal body weight
- PEEP

- FIO_2
- High-pressure limit alarm
- Percent minute ventilation (% Min. Vol.)

Based on the ideal body weight and the target minute volume, the ventilator will adapt the V_T, rate, pressure, I:E ratio, and mode based on the lung mechanics and pattern of breathing. If the patient is making little to no spontaneous effort, ASV applies volume-targeted pressure control. As the patient starts initiating more spontaneous breaths, ASV transitions from full support to partial support using pressure support breaths. The machine continues to adapt to the changing lung dynamics of the patient throughout all mode changes. Once the patient's tidal volume and respiratory rate meet the goals set, then ASV "backs off" and allows weaning.

Imagine if you set up adaptive support ventilation and enter the following:

IBW	60 kg
PEEP	5 cm H_20
FIO_2	40%
% Min. Vol.	100%

The ventilator will set a target minute volume of 6.0 liters. The ventilator in this mode sets a target volume of 100 cc/kg/min, thus 100 cc X 60 kg X 1.0 = 6000 cc or 6.0 L/min. If you set the % Min Vol. at 80%, the machine will change the target minute volume to 4.8 L/min (100 cc X 60 kg X .80 = 4800 cc or 4.8 L/min). The range in which you can set the % Min. Vol. is 50 to 350%.

Proportional Assist Ventilation (PAV)

Like pressure support and volume support, proportional assist ventilation is a spontaneous mode of ventilation, so the patient must be spontaneously breathing and have an intact respiratory drive. Basically, this mode works by setting the amount of work or effort you want the ventilator to provide, and the patient provides the rest. The range in which you can select is anywhere from 10 to 90%.

Therefore, if you set it up to 60% proportional assist, the ventilator will provide 60% of the work of breathing while the patient will have to provide the other 40%.

The machine knows how much inspiratory pressure or "effort" it needs to perform by taking constant measurements of the lungs' compliance and resistance. These measurements can change on a breath-to-breath basis, so if the patient is taking in a large breath one moment and a smaller breath the next, the machine automatically compensates for this.

The basic settings are:

- FIO_2 40 %
- PEEP 5 cm H_2O
- % Support 80 %

Synchronized Intermittent Mandatory Ventilation (SIMV)

This is probably the most commonly used mode in mechanical ventilation today. It is the first mode I discuss where the word "control" does not appear in the title. This means you are relinquishing some of your control and beginning to let the patient take control of her breathing. In other words, you are starting to allow the patient to "wean" off the ventilator.

To understand the concept of weaning, I sometimes compare it to someone who breaks a leg. For a while, the person should not bear weight on that leg. Eventually, they are able to do so. At this point, you do not take the crutches away as the patient is not ready and will most likely fall, potentially causing further harm. Mechanical ventilation is no different. When a patient is finally able to begin breathing on their own, you do not remove all support. You gradually lessen the support of the machine until the patient is ready to be removed from it all together. Sometimes, as in the case of post-op recovery, this process is relatively short. In other cases, such as trauma to the airways, this process can take quite a bit longer.

In SIMV, the fundamental change in the way you deliver mechanical ventilation is with regard to the spontaneous breaths. The first time the patient takes a spontaneous breath, it is no longer a controlled breath but instead a supported breath. A patient with a broken leg who is using crutches and walks without placing any weight on the injured leg is taking a controlled step. When the patient starts applying weight, the crutches are now providing a supported step. When you use this mode of ventilation, you will be using the same settings as previously discussed with the addition of one more setting. The additional setting is called pressure support. I will discuss the basic settings and explain how pressure support works. Here are the basic settings:

Tidal volume:	500 ml
Respiratory rate:	12 breaths/minute
F_IO_2:	40%
PEEP:	5 cm H_2O
Pressure support:	10 cm H_2O

With these settings, the patient will receive 12 breaths per minute with a tidal volume of 500 ml. This time, for each additional breath the patient takes, they will receive 10 cm H_2O of pressure support to help them with their inspiration. Spontaneous tidal volumes will vary depending on patient effort and the amount of pressure support that is set. *The pressure support will cycle on during the spontaneous inhalation cycle only.* It is not present during exhalation or during a machine-controlled breath. As the patient becomes stronger, you will begin to wean the pressure support and the number of machine-cycled breaths delivered to him or her. Some ventilators allow the SIMV mode to be used with volume, pressure, or PRVC to determine the type of machine-cycled breaths.

Pressure Support

In pressure support ventilation, there is no longer a set respiratory rate. All breaths taken are spontaneous breaths; therefore, no machine breaths are required. Each spontaneous breath is aided by the setting on the pressure support. An example of basic settings for pressure support is as follows:

Pressure support:	10 cm H_2O
F_IO_2:	40%
PEEP:	5 cm H_2O

This mode can be used *only* for a spontaneously breathing patient, and, as mentioned above, the pressure support is activated during the inhalation phase. PEEP is the only pressure that remains in the circuit upon exhalation.

Volume Support

Volume support ventilation works a little like PRVC. In volume support, a targeted tidal volume is set. The ventilator automatically adjusts the pressure support needed by the patient to achieve this volume.

Here are the basic settings:

Tidal volume:	500 ml
F_IO_2:	40%
PEEP:	5 cm H_2O

Like in pressure support, this mode can be used *only* for a spontaneously breathing patient.

Continuous Positive Airway Pressure (CPAP)

This mode can be done through invasive or non-invasive measures. An invasive measure means an intubated or trached patient. A non-invasive measure means the ventilation is delivered through a mask, creating a tight seal around the patient's nose and/or mouth. When a pressure is set, this pressure is the same throughout the breathing circuit during the inhalation and exhalation phase. This mode requires the patient to be spontaneously breathing. On most ventilators, CPAP is set with the PEEP button. PEEP is essentially the same as CPAP.

Here are the basic settings:

F_IO_2:	40%
CPAP/PEEP:	10 cm H_2O

BiPap

BiPap stands for two levels of positive airway pressure. Technically, it is the same as pressure support ventilation. Two levels of pressure are set: a higher level of pressure during the inhalation phase to augment the patient's spontaneous breathing and a lower level of pressure during the exhalation phase, allowing the patient to exhale easier against a lesser flow. The two settings are typically labeled as IPAP (Inspiratory Positive Airway Pressure) and EPAP (Expiratory Positive Airway Pressure).

Typical settings are as follows:

F_IO_2:	40%
IPAP:	10 cm H_2O
EPAP:	6 cm H_2O

Airway Pressure Release Ventilation (APRV)

APRV is an "open lung strategy" mode of ventilation. This means using a reverse inspiratory to expiratory ratio (I:E) to keep the lungs open for an extended duration followed by a short exhalation time for the purpose of removing CO_2. The patient is able to spontaneously breathe through the entire respiratory cycle.

Another way of looking at this mode is to realize that it is a modified form of CPAP. This mode is not meant for someone who is on paralytics. It is used on the spontaneously breathing patient and provides the added benefit of no paralytics and less sedation for the patient.

You may have also heard this mode called Bi-Vent™ or Bi-Level™, and because of the advanced nature of this mode, I will discuss it in greater detail. You will need to know the basic terminology used with this mode. Some of these terms might vary from ventilator to ventilator, but the meaning is still the same.

P High: The inspiratory pressure (similar to pressure control). It is usually set at 2 to 3 cm of pressure above the mean airway pressure the patient uses on the previous vent setting.

P Low: The same as PEEP, only it is labeled differently. It is the end expiratory pressure set on this mode. It is not used very often and is typically set at zero.

T High: This is basically the inspiratory time or the number of seconds during the inhalation phase. It is normally set at 3 to 4 seconds.

T Low: This is basically the expiratory time or the number of seconds during the exhalation phase. It is normally set at 0.6 to 0.8 seconds initially.

F_IO_2: The O_2 percentage the patient is receiving.

Let us assume these are the settings:

P High: 20 cm H_2O

P Low: 0 cm H_2O

T High: 4 seconds

T Low: 0.7 seconds

F_IO_2: 40%

Based on this information, the patient's lungs will be opened for 4 seconds at the set pressure of 20 cm H_2O. The exhalation phase will last 0.7 seconds before the inhalation phase will start over. The set respiratory rate for the patient in the APRV setting is calculated as such:

60 ÷ (T High + T Low)

60 ÷ (4 + 0.7) = 12.7 breaths/minute

PEEP is not set because you usually allow the patient to create their own intrinsic PEEP or auto PEEP. What is auto PEEP? Auto PEEP is created when the patient is on the mechanical ventilator, and you do not give them enough time to exhale before you start the next inhalation cycle. For example, you deliver a breath of 500 ml to a patient, and the patient is able to exhale only 480 ml before the next breath starts. There is still

20 ml of air in the lungs. This extra air produces a certain amount of pressure against the alveolar wall, creating auto PEEP. In APRV, you have a fairly short exhalation time, which allows the patient to create their own PEEP rather than actually setting the PEEP.

It is important that you always measure the auto PEEP to insure the patient is receiving the correct amount of PEEP. If the auto PEEP is too low, you risk greater pressure against the cardiovascular system, which can result in decreased cardiac output and decreased blood pressure.

I feel the need to discuss this mode in greater detail simply because it is more advanced and takes additional knowledge to operate. Remember, the information I am providing is the basic knowledge needed to understand these modes. *In no way does it qualify you to use these modes unless directed to do so by your employer.* I will now explain the settings used in ARV.

P High: I have already stated this number is usually set at 2 to 3 cm above the mean airway pressure from the previous setting. However, you can "fine tune" this number. If the delivered tidal volume is too low, one option you have to correct it is by increasing P High until the desired tidal volume or minute ventilation is achieved.

PEEP: As I have mentioned earlier, PEEP is usually not indicated in this mode. One exception where PEEP might be acceptable is when the lungs collapse quickly upon exhalation. An example where setting PEEP might be a good idea is when T Low (exhalation time) is set at 0.4 seconds, and the patient still has little or no auto PEEP.

T High: The initial setting, as mentioned before, is usually 3 to 4 seconds. By adjusting T High, either higher or lower, the set respiratory rate will also increase or decrease. By increasing T High, you will decrease the set rate, and by decreasing T High, you will increase the set rate. It is another way to alter the minute ventilation received from the patient. Depending on the I:E ratio, you may have to change T High by as much as 0.5 seconds to see a change in the overall respiratory rate.

T Low: By adjusting T Low, you are adjusting the exhalation time. The normal setting is 0.6 to 0.8 seconds; however, these numbers can vary greatly from patient to patient. One step that must be performed as soon as T Low is set is determining the auto PEEP. Each ventilator has a certain method to use in order to get the calculated auto PEEP. Usually, this consists of an inhalation pause followed quickly by an exhalation pause. Typically, you are shooting for a goal of 5 to 10 cm H_2O. In cases of COPD and other lung diseases, you may see a T Low as long as 1.5 seconds. If you continue to monitor the auto PEEP, then you may continue to increase T Low. You want to be careful, however, that you do not increase it too much and lose the reverse I:E ration, which allows APRV to be so beneficial. Remember, when you adjust T Low, the minute ventilation is also altered.

When T Low is increased, the amount of exhalation time increases, which means more air is exhaled, thus increasing minute ventilation. If you decrease T Low, the minute ventilation is decreased. By changing T Low by just 0.1 second, either up or down, it can create a fairly large change in the minute ventilation. This process is a fairly non-invasive way of altering your volume outcome.

Some ventilators that use this mode allow for the use of pressure support. Most often, pressure support is not needed. During the inspiratory phase of APRV, the lungs are already being held open by the amount of pressure set on P High. The higher this number, the longer the lungs are being held open. When a patient takes a spontaneous breath during the inspiratory phase, they will need only a very small breath to fill the remainder of the lungs. For this reason, the spontaneous tidal volume that is measured by the ventilator is usually a low number. It is common practice to add or increase pressure support when you see a small, spontaneous tidal volume; however, in this case, it is not necessary. In lower P High settings, it may be acceptable to add some pressure support. You must remember that the pressure support set will add to your total peak inspiratory pressure of the patient. The peak inspiratory pressure of a spontaneous breath during the inspiratory phase of APRV is calculated at the sum of P High and pressure support.

The three benefits of using the APRV mode of ventilation are as follows:

1. The longer inspiratory phase allows more time for gas exchange to occur at the alveolar level, thus increasing the PaO_2.

2. The longer inspiratory phase also helps to recruit additional alveoli.

3. The lungs are designed to reabsorb a certain amount of fluid. By holding the lungs open longer, you create a greater surface area, therefore allowing more fluid to be reabsorbed back into the lung tissue. This maneuver is beneficial to the fluid-overloaded patient.

High Frequency Ventilation

High frequency ventilation is considered a "non-conventional" mode of ventilation. As far as the level of understanding, it is an advanced mode, and it can be quite difficult to grasp its concepts. Basically, this mode uses an extremely high respiratory rate with an extremely low tidal volume to achieve ventilation. When in operation, it would appear that you are literally vibrating air into and out of the lungs due to this high rate.

High frequency ventilation should be considered when you have a patient on "conventional" modes of ventilation who is not receiving therapeutic benefits from this modality. In other words, the settings are at 100% F_IO_2, the peak pressure is greater than 30, and the PEEP is as high as you can go without negatively affecting the cardiac output.

The theory behind high frequency ventilation is that gas exchange can occur simply by the flow of air into and out of the lungs, given that the lungs are maintained in an open position. The peak airway pressure is relatively small, at times as low as 10 cm H_2O above baseline; however, with the high rate involved, the mean airway pressure can be comparative to that of "conventional" ventilation. Oxygenation occurs through the process of diffusion, thus the oxygen molecule must be in contact with the cellular wall in order for the process of diffusion to take place. By using a higher rate, there will be more opportunity for the oxygen molecule to have contact, therefore increasing the PAO_2.

Three types of high frequency ventilation exist today: high frequency positive pressure ventilation, high frequency jet ventilation, and high frequency oscillation.

High frequency positive pressure ventilation: Typically, the respiratory rate in this mode is set for 60 to 100 breaths/min with an I:E ratio of 1:3 or less. Tidal volumes are usually 20 to 30% of those found in traditional ventilation.

High frequency jet ventilation: The respiratory rate is a little higher, ranging from 100 to 200 breaths per minute. The I:E ratio is shortened to a 1:1 ratio, and the peak airway pressure is typically set at 8 to 10 cm H_2O above baseline.

High frequency oscillation: This mode appears to be a literal vibration of the chest as the respiratory rate dramatically increases from 60 to 3600 breaths per minute (1 to 60 Hertz). Reading about this mode cannot do it justice without actually observing it and witnessing its therapeutic benefits. With such a high respiratory rate, it has been shown that you actually increase the overall mean lung volume without a noticeable change in the mean airway pressure.

Neonatal/Pediatric Considerations

There are a few considerations that must be kept in mind as you shift your attention towards the care of the neonatal and pediatric population. The most obvious, of course, is the size of your patient. When dealing with such small lungs, your delivery method must be adjusted. There are many methods used when dealing with the ventilation of children. It is not my goal to discuss these methods but to provide you with a little understanding as to what modes are most commonly used and why.

Nasal CPAP is frequently used in the neonatal population. It is a noninvasive way of providing positive pressure through the nose in an attempt to avoid having to intubate the patient. The three most common indications for nasal CPAP are:

1) A spontaneously breathing baby that is in respiratory distress. This is evidenced by nasal flaring, retraction, and grunting.

2) PaO_2 is less than 60 with an F_IO_2 of .60 or greater.

3) When apnea spells are present.

Once the infant is intubated, the most common mode of ventilation would be a mode that is time-cycled and pressure limited, similar to the pressure control modes discussed previously. Time-cycled simply means an inspiratory and expiratory time are set. The machine will cycle each breath based on this time. Pressure limited means a peak inspiratory pressure is set for the machine to deliver. A neonate's lungs are much more delicate than those of an adult, thus you want to be sure not to use an excessively high pressure that could damage the lungs. Since the inspiratory pressure in volume ventilation varies with patient compliance, this mode may not be the best to use in this patient population. Again, in using the pressure limited mode, the minute ventilation will vary. Therefore, a greater amount of attention must be devoted to watching the machine to insure that the patient is never under ventilated based on a change in the compliance of the lungs.

High frequency ventilation is a strategy used more in the infant population rather than the adult population. If the infant is not being oxygenated and/or ventilated appropriately with traditional ventilator modes on high settings, this mode may be an option to consider.

The last strategy to discuss Is Extracorporeal Membrane Oxygenation (ECMO). ECMO is not a mode of ventilation. It is a process that bypasses the lungs. In ECMO the venous blood is removed, usually from the right jugular vein, and sent through a machine that oxygenates respiratory rate dramatically increases from 60 to 3600 breaths per minute (1 to 60 Hertz). Reading about this mode cannot do it justice without actually observing it and witnessing its therapeutic benefits. With such a high respiratory rate, it has been shown that you actually increase the overall mean lung volume without a noticeable change in the mean airway pressure.

the blood through a membrane. The blood is then returned to the body. Bypassing the heart and lungs provides an opportunity for these organs to rest. ECMO is usually reserved for the critically ill child who is in some type of reversible respiratory or cardiac failure.

As the infant grows and enters the pediatric population, the modes of ventilation are basically the same as with the adult population. The respiratory rates and tidal volumes are lower due to the physical nature of the child's lungs. As the child grows and matures, the means of treatment become closer to that of an adult.

Ventilator Alarms

What would the I.C.U. be without alarms? Some people may view alarms as a nuisance that must be endured during a shift; however, as you all know, alarms are an important indication that something is not right. It is vital that you understand ventilator alarms: what they mean, how they should be set, and hot to correct the problem that is being identified. With such a variety of ventilators are on the market, there is a plethora of alarms that exist that you may never encounter. I will cover the most common alarms that everyone should know and be aware of.

High pressure: Measured in cm of H_2O and is usually set at about 10 cm of H_2O above the peak airway pressure that the patient is achieving based on the current ventilator settings. It is important to have this alarm set at the appropriate level. In most ventilators, inspiration will stop once it achieves this value, thus protecting the lungs from dangerously high peak airway pressures that could cause damage such as barotrauma.

Several causes can produce a high peak airway pressure such as: decreased lung compliance, increased secretions, bronchoconstriction, and kinking of the circuit or E.T. Tube. These problems can usually be corrected by suctioning the airway, administering a bronchodialator, or removing the kink from the circuit.

Low pressure: Measured in cm of H_2O and is usually set at about 10 cm of H_2O below the peak airway pressure that the patient is achieving based on the current ventilator settings. When this alarm sounds, it is most likely an indication the patient has become disconnected from the ventilator or a significant leak has occurred within the circuit. Starting with the patient and working back towards the ventilator, check the entire circuit until you find the leak and/or disconnect and correct the problem. The other possibility is the patient may have become extubated. Remember, when trying to identify a problem, always start with the patient and then proceed to the equipment.

Apnea alarms: This alarm may show on the ventilator screen as "BACKUP VENTILATION" and is usually set at 20 seconds. If the patient goes longer than 20 seconds without taking or receiving a breath, the machine will alarm. Most ventilators have backup settings that will activate at this point to ensure the patient is being adequately ventilated. This alarm will usually occur when the patient is in pressure support ventilation and has stopped breathing.

Low volume: This alarm can either mean low tidal volume or low minute ventilation depending on the ventilator. Either way, it is an indication that the patient is not receiving the volume of air that you would like to achieve. There is no "gold standard" as to where these alarms should be set. For example the minute ventilation alarm is usually set at 2-5 l/min below the minute ventilation that the patient is achieving. The problem is usually patient disconnect from the ventilator or a leak in the ciurcuit. Again, follow the circuit starting at the patient and work your way through until you identify the problem.

High respiratory rate: This alarm sounds when the patient is breathing above the value set for the high rate. This problem could be patient discomfort either from pain or ventilator settings. Be sure the patient is adequately sedated or make ventilator changes that would be more comfortable for the patient. Many people ask what changes are appropriate. There is no patent answer to this question. Every patient is different. You will need to test various settings until you find what works best for your patient at that time. Another possible cause could be water in the circuit. If the ventilator is attached to a heated humidifier, water or condensation may form in the tubing. If too much water collects and begins to bubble as air moves through the circuit, the ventilator may misinterpret the bubbling for attempts to breathe by the patient. Simply draining the water from the circuit will correct the problem.

Low gas source: Ventilators are connected to compressed air and oxygen sources either from a tank or piped in through the wall. These sources run at 50 pounds per square inch, which is the pressure needed to run most ventilators. If the ventilator becomes disconnected from the wall, this alarm will sound. Simply reconnect the gas source. If the ventilator is still attached to the gas source, something more serious has occurred. There is a problem with the incoming gas source. The ventilator must be connected to an oxygen tank until maintenance can correct the problem.

Basic Ventilator Changes That Affect Blood Gas Values

In the world of mechanical ventilation, you have the ability to make ventilator changes which can alter the arterial blood gas readings. When looking at blood gas values, the only two you can directly affect are the CO_2 and PaO_2. Indirectly, the HCO_3^- level can also be affected but only as a compensatory mechanism. This leaves you with trying to correct and/or adjust the CO_2 and the PaO_2 levels.

If the PaO_2 levels are low and all of the other values are normal then you have a few options to try and correct this issue. I have listed a few of the more common corrective measures below:

1) Increase the FIO_2: This is usually the most obvious answer; however, given the fact that high levels of oxygen does carry with it a risk to our patient it is not usually the first option I would choose.
2) Increase PEEP: This will hold or "trap" more air in the lungs upon exhalation creating an increased mean airway pressure. Increasing the mean airway pressure increase the opportunity for gas exchange to take place. The biggest risk to high level of PEEP would be that of cardiovascular side effects. Anytime you are making a ventilator change it is essential to monitor the patient's hemodynamic status. If it declines after an adjustment such as an

increase in PEEP, then it is quite possible that the higher pressure is impeding the cardiovascular system.

3) Increasing the inspiratory time: By having a higher inspiratory time you are essentially holding the oxygen molecule in the airways for a slightly greater period of time. The more time it is in contact with the alveolar wall, the greater the opportunity for gas exchange to take place.
4) Increase the tidal volume: This can be done in volume modes by simply increasing the set tidal volume, in pressure modes it would be done by increasing the set inspiratory pressure. It is possible that if the tidal volume breath was not large enough than the oxygen may not have been getting far enough into the airway to reach the area of gas exchange.

CO_2 is controlled through the amount of minute ventilation from the patient. Minute ventilation is calculated by multiplying the respiratory rate X the tidal volume. If the CO_2 is too high, then you must increase the minute ventilation to "blow off" more CO_2. If the CO_2 is too low, then the patient is being over ventilated. This can be corrected by decreasing the minute ventilation. Again I have listed a few of the more common corrective measures below:

1) Increase the tidal volume: Done as mentioned above.
2) Increase the respiratory rate
3) Decrease PEEP: If the oxygenation is doing well then decreasing PEEP can help remove CO_2. A decrease in PEEP will allow more air to escape during exhalation.

4) Increasing inspiratory time: Sometimes a high CO_2 level has nothing to do with minute ventilation. I have seen minute ventilations as high as 17 lpm with a resulting high CO_2. That is simply air moving in and out of the lung. If gas exchange is not occurring at the alveolar level then all the air moving and out is not going to help the situation. By having an increased inspiratory time will not only help improve gas exchange for oxygen, but it will also help gas exchange as it relates to carbon dioxide.

No matter what choice you make to attempt and correct the abnormality none of it will do any good if you don't identify what is causing the problem. In fact, the first step should be to identify what is causing the problem. This can help us determine the best course of action to take to treat the patient. Again, the list of abnormalities is extensive. There are volumes of textbooks devoted to this topic alone. Listed next are some of the more common issues:

- The patient may be bronchoconstricted in which case a bronchodilator may help.
- The patient may have a mucus plug thus requiring suctioning.
- The patient may have COPD or other underlying pulmonary condition.
- The patient may have trauma to the lungs such as a pulmonary contusion, multiple rib fractures, hemothorax, or pneumothorax.
- The patient may have developed a serious pulmonary complication known as ARDS (Acute Respiratory Distress Syndrome).
- They may be fluid overloaded creating pulmonary edema.
- They may have a pulmonary embolism.

If you ask 100 different doctors what ventilator changes they would make to improve a patient's status you may not get 100 different answers, but I'm willing to bet you will quite a few different answers. The same goes for what ventilator mode is the best and what is the best way to "wean" someone from the ventilator. My goal here is to get you into the game of understanding where it all comes from. In the end you must do what is commonly accepted practice where you work.

Blood Gas Interpretation

An arterial blood gas (ABG) is a lab test that produces the following critical information: PaO_2 (oxygen), $PaCO_2$ (carbon dioxide), HCO_3- (bicarbonate), and pH. The blood is drawn from an artery that can measure these values *before* the blood enters the tissues of the body, at which time values can be altered.

When obtaining an arterial blood gas, it is important to insure that you are providing a good sample to the lab. The syringe must be a heparanized syringe to prevent the sample form clotting. The collected sample must be free of air bubbles and quickly delivered to the lab. As soon as the blood is drawn, the values can start changing due to metabolism.

It is essential to understand the basics of arterial blood gas interpretation and to know how ventilator changes can affect the outcome of blood gas. In this section, I will explain what you will need to know in order to have a solid foundation.

As in the mechanical ventilation portion of this book, there are several definitions you will need to learn before continuing:

Acidemia: Occurs when the measured pH is less than 7.35.

Acidosis: A patient condition that causes academia, such as increased CO_2 or decreased HCO_3-.

Alkalemia: Occurs when the measured pH in the blood is greater than 7.45.

Alkalosis: A patient condition that causes alkalemia, such as decreased CO_2 or increased HCO_3-.

Hypoxemia: A PaO_2 that is less than normal in arterial blood.

Hypoxia: A decreased level of oxygen in the tissues.

HCO_3-: A measurement showing the level of bicarbonate in the blood. Bicarbonate is a buffer found in blood, helping to alter the pH level. This is measured in mEq/L.

PaO_2: The partial pressure of oxygen found in the arterial blood. It is measured in mm Hg.

$PaCO_2$: The partial pressure of carbon dioxide found in the arterial blood. It is measured in mm Hg.

pH: The measure of the acid/base balance found in blood.

NORMAL ABG VALUES	
pH	7.35 – 7.45
$PaCO_2$	35 – 45 mm Hg
HCO_3-	22 – 26 mEq/L
PaO_2	80 – 100 mm Hg

I have not yet discussed the base excess, a value you may see in your blood gas values. The normal value for base excess is -2 to +2, with 0 being ideal. Some institutions use base excess rather than HCO_3-, and there is an ongoing debate over which value is better. For the purpose of this review, rather than writing at length about this debate, I will be using all examples with HCO_3- as my value. Be sure to check with your employer as to which value is being used at your facility.

The Process of ABG Interpretation

Step 1: pH Classification

This is one of the most critical numbers that you should review regarding the blood gas. You must determine if the patient is within normal limits, acidemic, or alkalemic. As previously mentioned, the normal pH is 7.35 to

7.45. If the pH is greater than 7.45, the patient is considered alkalemic. If the pH is less than 7.35, the patient is considered acidemic.

Step 2: $PaCO_2$ Classification

The normal range for $PaCO_2$ is 35 to 45 mm Hg. If the CO_2 is greater than 45, the patient is considered acidotic. If the CO_2 is less than 35, the patient is considered alkalotic. CO_2 affects the pH in an inverse relationship. If the CO_2 increases, the pH will decrease. If the CO_2 decreases, the pH will increase. The pH may also be within normal limits, but remember, you can be acidotic without being acidemic. Acidosis is the condition in which leads to acidemia. The proper terminology for an abnormal CO_2 value is either respiratory alkalosis or respiratory acidosis.

$\uparrow$ ventilation = $\downarrow$ $PaCO_2$

$\downarrow$ ventilation = $\uparrow$ $PaCO_2$

Step 3: HCO_3- Classification

The normal range for HCO_3- is 22 to 26 mEq/L. If the HCO_3- is greater than 26, the patient has an alkalotic condition. If the HCO_3- is less than 22, the patient has an acidotic condition. HCO_3- affects the pH in a direct relationship. If the HCO_3- increases, the pH will also increase. If the HCO_3- decreases, the pH will decrease as well. The proper terminology for an abnormal HCO_3- is either metabolic alkalosis or metabolic acidosis.

Step 4: Determine if the condition is compensated or uncompensated

Our bodies are structured in such a way that if something goes wrong, it will often try to correct the problem. If the body finds itself in an acidotic or alkalotic situation, it will try to compensate through the opposite mechanism that caused the problem. For example, if the problem is related to respiratory, the kidneys will either expel the HCO_3- or retain it in an effort to bring the pH within normal range. If the problem is metabolic-related, the breathing pattern will change in such a way as to either eliminate more CO_2 or retain it in an effort to correct the abnormal pH.

There are three categories in which the patient can belong: uncompensated, partially compensate, or fully compensated.

Uncompensated is a condition in which the pH is abnormal, but the body has made no attempt to correct it. For example, the pH is low and the CO_2 is high indicating a respiratory acidosis. The HCO_3^- is within normal limits; therefore, no compensation by the body is present. Uncompensated conditions usually represent an acute change.

Partially compensated is a condition in which the pH is still abnormal; however, the body has begun to make changes in an attempt to correct the problem. Again, you have a respiratory acidosis;

but, this time, when you look at the HCO_3^-, it has risen above the normal range in an attempt to correct the pH.

Fully compensated is a condition in which the pH is within normal limits and both the CO_2 and HCO_3^- are out-of-range. Using respiratory acidosis as an example, the pH is normal, and the CO_2 and HCO_3^- are elevated. The Hco_3^- has increased to a point in which the pH was brought back to a normal level. Fully compensated conditions usually represent a chronic change.

Step 5: Evaluate the PaO_2

The normal range for PaO_2 is 80 – 100 mm Hg. For levels below 80, the patient is considered to be hypoxemic, and additional oxygen may be required. For patients on supplemental oxygen, you may see a value higher than 100. In this case, you can start to wean the level of oxygen they are receiving.

BLOOD GAS EXAMPLES

1.	pH	7.41
	$PaCO_2$	43 mm Hg
	HCO_3^-	24 mEq/L
	PaO_2	88 mm Hg

Interpretation: A normal blood gas.

2. pH 7.32

$PaCO_2$ 49 mm Hg

HCO_3^- 25 mEq/L

PaO_2 84 mm Hg

The pH is low indicating acidemia. The $PaCO_2$ is high indicating acidosis. The HCO_3^- is normal; therefore, no compensation has occurred. The PaO_2 is within normal limits.

Interpretation: Uncompensated respiratory acidosis.

3. pH 7.48

$PaCO_2$ 32 mm Hg

HCO_3^- 22 mEq/L

PaO_2 76 mm Hg

The pH is high indicating alkalemia. The $PaCO_2$ is low indicating alkalosis. The HCO_3^- is normal showing no compensation has occurred. The PaO_2 is low indicating the patient is also hypoxemic.

Interpretation: Uncompensated respiratory alkalosis.

4. pH 7.30

$PaCO_2$ 51 mm Hg

HCO_3^- 27 mEq/L

PaO_2 69 mm Hg

The pH is low indicating acidemia. The $PaCO_2$ is high indicating acidosis. The HCO_3^- is also high showing there is some level of compensation. Since the pH is still not within normal limits you only have a partial compensation. The PaO_2 is low; therefore, the patient is hypoxemic.

Interpretation: Partially compensated respiratory acidosis.

5. pH 7.49

$PaCO_2$ 30 mm Hg

HCO_3^- 19 mEq/L

PaO_2 74 mm Hg

The pH is high indicating alkalemia. The $PaCO_2$ is low indicating alkalosis. The HCO_3^- is also low showing there is some compensation; however, since the pH is still not within normal limits, it is only a partial compensation. The PaO_2 is low; therefore, the patient is hypoxemic.

Interpretation: Partially compensated respiratory alkalosis.

6. pH 7.35

$PaCO_2$ 50 mm Hg

HCO_3^- 29 mEq/L

PaO_2 78 mm Hg

The pH is normal. The $PaCO_2$ is high indicating acidosis. The HCO_3^- is high showing the patient is compensating. Since the pH is within normal limits, you have a fully compensated situation. The PaO_2 is low; therefore, the patient is hypoxemic.

Interpretation: Fully compensated respiratory acidosis.

7. pH 7.45

$PaCO_2$ 30 mm Hg

HCO_3^- 20 mEq/L

PaO_2 75 mm Hg

The pH is normal. The $PaCO_2$ is low indicating alkalosis. The HCO_3^- is also low showing there is compensation occurring. Since the pH is within normal limits, this gas is fully compensated. The PaO_2 is low; therefore, the patient is hypoxemic.

Interpretation: Fully compensated respiratory alkalosis.

8. pH 7.30

$PaCO_2$ 40 mm Hg

HCO_3^- 15 mEq/L

PaO_2 60 mm Hg

The pH is low indicating acidemia. The $PaCO_2$ is normal. The HCO_3^- is low indicating acidosis. The PaO_2 is low; therefore, the patient is hypoxemic.

Interpretation: Uncompensated metabolic acidosis.

9. pH 7.48

$PaCO_2$ 40 mm Hg

HCO_3^- 28 mEq/L

PaO_2 80 mm Hg

The pH is high indicating alkalemia. The $PaCO_2$ is normal. The HCO_3^- is high indicating alkalosis. The PaO_2 is normal.

Interpretation: Uncompensated metabolic alkalosis.

10. pH 7.28

$PaCO_2$ 32 mm Hg

HCO_3^- 18 mEq/L

PaO_2 75 mm Hg

The pH is low indicating acidemia. The $PaCO_2$ is decreased creating an alkalotic situation. The patient is not alkalotic indicating there must be some level of compensation occurring. However, only partial compensation is occurring since the pH is still not within normal limits. The HCO_3^- is low indicating acidosis. The PaO_2 is low; therefore, the patient is hypoxemic.

Interpretation: Partially compensated metabolic acidosis.

11. pH 7.54

$PaCO_2$ 49 mm Hg

HCO_3^- 32 mEq/L

PaO_2 88 mm Hg

The pH is high indicating alkalemia. The $PaCO_2$ is increased which should produce an acidotic condition. The patient is not acidemic; therefore, some level of compensation is occurring. The HCO_3^- is high indicating alkalosis. The PaO_2 is within normal limits.

Interpretation: Partially compensated metabolic alkalosis.

12. | | |
|---|---|
| pH | 7.35 |
| $PaCO_2$ | 30 mm Hg |
| HCO_3^- | 19 mEq/L |
| PaO_2 | 90 mm Hg |

The pH is normal. The $PaCO_2$ is low indicating alkalosis. The HCO_3^- is low indicating acidosis. The PaO_2 is within normal limits.

Interpretation: Fully compensated metabolic acidosis.

13. pH 7.44

$PaCO_2$ 51 mm Hg

HCO_3^- 17 mEq/L

PaO_2 58 mm hg

The pH is normal. The $PaCO_2$ is high indicating acidosis. The HCO_3^- is high indicating alkalosis. The PaO_2 is low; therefore, the patient is hypoxemic.

Interpretation: Fully compensated metabolic alkalosis.

14. pH 7.28

$PaCO_2$ 56 mm Hg

HCO_3^- 17 mEq/L

PaO_2 52 mm Hg

The pH is low indicating acidemia. The $PaCO_2$ is high indicating acidosis. The HCO_3^- is low indicating acidosis. The PaO_2 is low; therefore, the patient is hypoxemic.

Interpretation: Combination of metabolic and respiratory acidosis.

15. pH 7.52

$PaCO_2$ 32 mm Hg

HCO_3^- 30 mEq/L

PaO_2 66 mm Hg

The pH is high indicating alkalemia. The $PaCO_2$ is low indicating alkalosis. The HCO_3^- is high indicating alkalosis. The PaO_2 is low; therefore the patient is hypoxemic.

Interpretation: Combination metabolic and respiratory alkalosis.

CHECK OUT OTHER TITLES BY THIS AUTHOR AT:

WWW.MICHAELFISCHERAUTHOR.COM

Made in the USA
Las Vegas, NV
23 October 2023